My Kind of Yoga™

TEACHER TRAINING MANUAL

Ann-See Yeoh *BA(Hons) MMedSci*

Copyright ©2021 Ann-See Yeoh

ISBN: 978-1-9196086-0-0

Setting your Intention for the Programme

Prepare

Be open and ready to embark on this journey

Set your Intention

What is your Intention for this training programme?

Select and Decide

We will be covering lots of information; some new, some not, some applicable right now, some are not. Make notes, ask questions, sieve the information and apply it appropriately

Breathe

There will be highs and lows on this journey.   Relax and breathe.

Piece it together

Understand the pieces of the puzzle here. Practice and the pieces will fall into place.

Listen to your body

Make sure you are comfortable in the learning environment. Sit, lay down, stretch and move your body.

Self-reflection

Contemplate what we learn, discuss and discover here on, and off, the mat

Introduction

The human body is not an instrument to be used, but a realm of one's being to be experimented, explored, enriched and, thereby, educated.

THOMAS HANNA

I came to yoga many years ago and in 2003, I reached a place of development of my ideas for both yoga philosophy and alignment technique that was relevant to my personal needs, as well as those who come to yoga from the fitness world. So, back then, I created Pathway to Yoga, as an introduction to the more traditional yoga forms and as the name suggests, provides participants with a pathway into the world of yoga using the physical Poses (ĀSANA).

This course ran successfully for numerous years and came to a halt when my work emphasis changed and my business partner moved back to Portugal. During that time, I was also undergoing my yoga teacher training course and as life unfolded around me, I took stock of what I was doing and decided to consolidate what I was doing and what was important to me at that time.

I sincerely value the wisdom that my teachers have shared with me and I look to integrate their wisdom, and the wisdom of yoga, into my everyday life. I wanted to share my love and experience of yoga with those who are inspired to do the same. Yoga has touched my heart and life and has become who I am and what I want to contribute to humanity.

The materials presented in this manual represent a personal composition and interpretation of yoga. Yoga is both a science and an art of a deeper understanding of the human condition. Yoga is a practice of revelation, a revelation of who you really are.

I believe that we are inherently the same; yet, we wear differences, differences in body shape, physical ability, mental focus, mental toughness, spiritual development, human evolvement. Hence, yoga practice is about getting you to find your own yoga, getting the yoga to fit the individual rather than the other way around.

I believe that every time you take a deep, conscious breath you have experienced yoga.

I believe that, as with any sharing of knowledge, each individual takes that knowledge, adds it to their model of the world, and moulds that new found knowledge to suit their view.

Hence, the birth of My Kind of Yoga™.

Welcome to your journey.

I am honoured and blessed to help guide you on your way.

Be blessed. Be happy.

Namaste.

What is Yoga?

Yoga is a way of moving into stillness in order to experience the truth of who you are.

ERICH SCHIFFMAN

Yoga is the current of spirituality that has developed on the Indian peninsula over a period of some five thousand years. Over the years, yoga has assumed various forms. However, underlying all forms of yoga is the understanding that the human being is more than the physical body and that, through practice, it is possible to discover what this "more" is.

Yoga entered the West mainly through the missionary work of Swami Vivekananda, who spoke at the Parliament of Religions in 1893. His message of tolerance and compassion to all living things was received with a standing ovation.

The twentieth century saw a continued movement of wisdom from India to the West. The most influential yogi of all was Tirumalai Krishnamacharya. Krishnamacharya was a master of yoga, Ayurveda, Sanskrit, and Logic. He was responsible for creating Ashtanga Vinyasa Yoga, teaching Pattabhi Jois, who continued to teach this style throughout his life, as well as B.K.S. Iyengar, Indra Devi, and his own son Desikachar. Krishnamacharya himself never crossed an ocean, but his influence is responsible for the incredible spread of asana practice in the West. He was the first Brahmin to teach a woman yoga, and a western woman at that. He lived to be 101 years old, still vital and teaching even late in life.

The yoga we are familiar with in the West is largely physical. The arrival of Astanga Vinyasa Yoga, with its intensity, heat, and level of difficulty appealed, and still appeals, to body-conscious practitioners. For many people, this practice in its entirety is impossible to perform based on bone structure limitations. For this reason, many teachers began to teach Power Yoga, or a flow-based derivative of Astanga Yoga based on the idea of "Vinyasa"–the linking of one posture to the next using breath and movement.

As yoga continues to grow in popularity, it is also evolving. The move from East to West is leading to a loss of its original cultural and religious context. We are at a point in the evolution of this practice of yoga where we are able to apply the magnificent teachings of the past to our present situation.

The yoga practice will adapt itself; it always has.

It is up to us to create meaning within the practice that is appropriate to our present situation.

Brief Historical Timeline

3500 BCE	The first time the term "yoga" appears in any literature, i.e. the Rig Veda
1000 BCE	In the Atharva Veda, yoga is related to the pranayama practiced by priests
800 BCE	Yoga appears in the Upanishads
300 BCE	The Maitri (or Maitrayani) Upanishad gives the first fully developed system of yoga. The Maitri Upanishad defines six limbs of yoga (sadanga) as control of the breath (pranayama), withdrawal of the senses (pratyahara), meditation (dhyana), concentration (dharana), contemplation (tarka) and absorption (samadhi). This Upanishad goes on to describe liberation (kaivalya) as the restraint of thoughts and absorption in self-luminous witness consciousness. These are all the core concepts and practices that we see in the Yoga Sutras.
100 BCE	Patanjali wrote the Yoga Sutras. To the Maitri sadanga are added restraints (yama), observances (niyama) and posture (asana). Tarka is dropped from the set giving us eight limbs (astanga).
1300	Svatmarama produced Hatha Yoga Pradipika, a tantric text describing sixteen asanas; variants of Padmasana. Note that these are all seated postures, specifically for pranayama and meditation, for attainment of samadhi. It is 1,500 years after Patanjali that yoga begins to be associated with asana.
1893	Swami Vivekenanda spoke at the Parliament of Religions. Since then, Yoga has undergone a unique metamorphosis. In the hands of numerous Western Yoga teachers, most of who have learned (Hatha) Yoga from other Westerner teachers rather than native Indian gurus, YOga has been tailored to suit the specific needs of their respective countrymen and women.

My Kind of Yoga™

My Kind of Yoga™ is an Intentional Movement System that allows you to explore your internal landscape. Intention has to do with heart. The power of the heart is the driving force behind all and what we do; in yoga and in life. Movement is about what we do with our body. The beauty of the human body in action, when moving with intention and awareness is a wondrous thing. It's not about the shapes you can create with your body. It's about the feel and what you can create within that makes your practice beautiful.

ANN-SEE YEOH

My Kind of Yoga™ is a a culmination of my life experiences. It is a simple, straightforward approach to yoga. It is about self-exploration and is a journey of personal discovery.

Anatomically and physiologically, we are different. Genetically, you could argue that we are the same, but in terms of how our bodies function, and how our mind works, we are different.

What distinguishes My Kind of Yoga™ as a Practice is a 2-step approach:

1. The Practice

2. The Play

The Practice

My Kind of Yoga™ is all about the participant and empowering them to practice their kind of yoga. Each Practice will have different intentions, and will have set sections.

The typical My Kind of Yoga™ Practice is:

1. Earth, where we get settled and grounded.

2. Water, where we begin to flow, get warm and ready to move

3. Fire, where we bring heat to all levels of the person, mind, body, energetically.

4. Air, where we begin to fall and focus on breath

5. Space, where we rest

The Play

As already mentioned, we are different anatomically and physiologically. For this reason, the Poses and the Practice should be modified to suit the individual, and so you would take into account physical ability, fitness levels, any existing injuries, joint issues, diseases, illnesses, etc.

What we should also consider is everyone's physical and mental condition is forever changing. You could wake up one morning with a stiff neck and another with pain in your shoulder. One afternoon, you may have lots of energy, or you may be recovering from the flu. The same applies for the people who come to our classes.

With all this in mind, we can encourage a sense of Play on the mat and through Play, modifying the Poses helps keep it interesting and help our participants stay present throughout the Practice. And, we encourage Play through being very self-aware of the body, breath and mind-set.

The Science behind My Kind of Yoga™

This is the basis of putting together a My Kind of Yoga™ class. Whilst you will learn and get to grips with three My Kind of Yoga™ Practices on this course, understanding the general principles behind the thought process will help you appreciate why the Poses are linked together in the way they are. It will also help you decide on how to adapt the Practice and/or the Poses to suit your class better, and it will give you the understanding in order to create your own Practices.

These principles are the fundamental building blocks, and with a deep understanding of them, you will be able to deviate away from them to create something that flows for you.

The principles are:

1. **Prepare** for the Lesson

2. Decide on the **Lesson Plan**

3. Mindfully **Lead** your class

4. **Self-reflect** on your teaching

1 Prepare

In order to create an appropriate space and environment for our participants, we need to consider a number of things. These include:

- The physical space we will be holding the class

- Our understanding of our participants

- Our head space

Create the Space

It is possible to practice Yoga anywhere. Yet, we can identify certain environmental conditions that are favourable to the Practice. In terms of teaching, you need to know where and who you are going to do teach.

SO, LET US BRAINSTORM. WHERE WILL YOU BE TEACHING AND TO WHOM?

Knowing Your Participants

Once you know the environment in which you will be holding the class, knowing your participants will help you decide on the lesson plan to use, and how to adapt the lesson to suit.

WHAT ARE SOME THINGS YOU WOULD CONSIDER?

Getting in the right head space

It is crucial to consider your head space and emotional state before teaching a class. The energy you bring to class will affect the class, as you are holding the space. We need to be open, centred and in a good space (SUKHA).

SO, WHAT MAY YOU WANT TO CONSIDER?

2 Decide on the Lesson Plan

Depending on your class, have a look at the Lesson Plans that have been provided and select the one most appropriate for your class. Each month, you will receive a new lesson plan.

Once you have selected a lesson plan, it is best to stick to the one lesson plan for a month. This allows your class participants to get stuck into the Practice and the Poses. Most people tend to come to class once a week, so they will need more than 4 sessions to get the feel of the Poses and the Intention of the Practice in their bodies and minds.

Each class is different and will need to be taught in a different way. You can do a certain amount of preparation beforehand by deciding if you are going to use the Lesson Plan in its entirety, or if you are going to break it down over the month. Stick with the Lesson Plan. Where you can vary it in the transitions between Poses, how you break the Sequence/ Blocks down, and/or how you add to them.

WHAT ARE SOME THINGS YOU COULD CONSIDER WHEN CHOOSING A LESSON PLAN?

Understanding the Intention for the Practice

The intention for the class is what you and your class focus on; it is your outcome, or objective. What are you wanting your class to achieve from a particular practice?

The intention can be something tangible, that focuses on the physical body, e.g. opening the hips, strengthening the upper body, lengthening the hamstrings. It could also be intangible, e.g. grounding, calming, heart opening. The choices here are limited only by your imagination. The tangible stuff is easier to play with. The intangible stuff is where the fun lies.

On this training programme, you will come away with three Practices, each with a different Intention. Ongoing, you will have access to a backlog of Practices and further Practices each month.

The Intention you choose to focus on will influence which lesson plan you choose. Select the practice that will enhance the Intention.

You can choose to focus on an intention for the month, or change it weekly, or even daily. By having a monthly intention, it gives your participants time to get stuck in, especially if the intention is something you are looking for them to take off the mat and into their daily life. Behaviour change takes time, which is why most traditional yoga courses run over the course of a couple of years or so. Doing the physical practice is one thing; even then we know it takes time to develop strength and to become more flexible. Living the philosophy takes even more time, especially if they are only practicing yoga once a week.

Encouraging the right attitude and will, are key to fulfilling the Intention. The stronger the Intention, the greater the cultivation of willpower.

Opening the Class

Earth

Most people, upon arriving for class, will need some time to settle and centre themselves. So, allow approximately 5 minutes to help them do that.

Timing	Pose	Teaching Points
1-3 minutes	Easy Sitting / Mountain / Corpse	• Allow them to get comfortable. • Check in with body • Check in with head space • Check in with emotions, energy • Take time to breathe • Introduce Locational Breathing
4-5 minutes	Gentle movement with breath, e.g. if sitting, tilt neck, simple seated twist. If standing, raise and lower arms, a few times, them move into Standing Forward Fold	• Guide them to compare right and left sides of the body • Slow, mindful breathing as they move to allow them to notice how the movements feel • Asking them to close their eyes is useful to draw their attention inwards

Water

Once they have settled, we start to flow even more to warm the body and breath.

Timing	Pose	Teaching Points
5 minutes	Sun Salutation	• Guide them through one round of the Sun Salutation visually as well as verbally • If they need to guidance, physically go through another round, this time teaching when to breathe and the name of the Pose • If they have it, stop demonstrating the sequence yourself; walk around, observe whilst still cueing the breath/Pose • Allow them at least 2 rounds on their own

Closing the Class

The Close of the Class is the icing on the cake, so it is worth taking the time to think about how you are going to finish the class. People want to feel good when they leave; they want to feel "complete", and that comes down to you listening to your gut instinct to some degree.

For the typical one-hour class, you are looking at getting your class to spend no more than 10 minutes lying down at the end of class. Too long, and lethargy sets in, and remember that the whole point of Yoga practice is to get energy to flow well.

WHAT SHOULD YOU CONSIDER WHEN CLOSING THE CLASS?

Space

Releasing both mental and physical tension can bring many benefits, including the lowering of blood pressure, reducing the risk of coronary heart disease, improving quality of sleep, and a certain degree of chronic and acute pain relief, and other psychosomatic disorders. Relaxation is not Meditation. It is about bringing the body to a rested state.

With a 60-minute class, we tend to allocate a maximum of 10 minutes for this part of the class. When we spend too long here, lethargy will set in, which counteracts the benefits of yoga practice.

Whilst there are many Relaxation methods, follow the steps below:

- Where possible, dim or turn off, any bright lights

- Get your participants to adopt a comfortable position, ideally lying in Corpse Pose

- You may wish to:

    - Tie in your Intention for the Relaxation with your Intention from your Practice. This Intention should be short and positively phrased and is intended to reshape behaviour and thought process. Repeat it three times. It should not be changed until it is achieved and the exact wording should be used on each occasion.

    - Settle in to your choice of Relaxation

- At the end of this section, bring your participants out of this deep rested state gradually by practising awareness of breath. You may with to repeat your Intention.

3 Mindfully Lead your Class

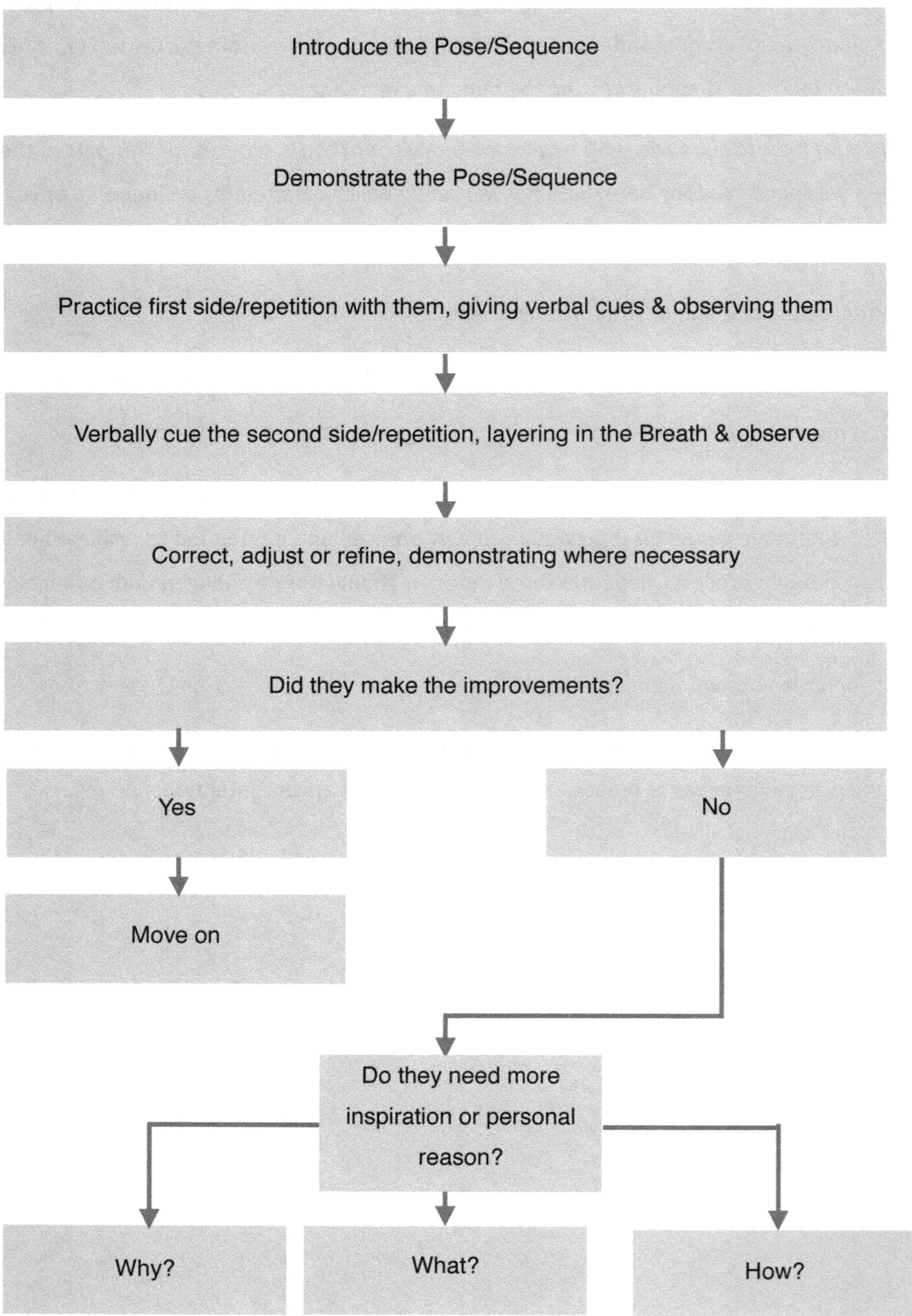

Organising your Thoughts

It is helpful to arrange your thoughts, cues, demonstrations, observations and adjustments according to three categories:

1. **Shape:** The shape of the Pose. With My Kind of Yoga™, we want our class participants to explore the Poses and establish what works for them, so it is not necessary to have each participant practice the classical form of the Pose. Do however, have a very clear image in your mind about how you want their Poses to look, and how to get into and out of it.

2. **Safety:** As their guide, we have to help our class participants stay safe in the Pose. Remind them about common misalignments and how to avoid them.

3. **SHRI:** SHRI means "beauty" or "refined expression", so find ways of helping them go deeper into a Pose and refine their expression of the Pose. This is only appropriate when Shape and Safety are established.

Demonstrating the Pose/Sequence

Humans are visual creatures. Most of us process information based on what we see. According to the Social Science Research Network, 65% of us are visual learners. Therefore, it is important to consider your position in the class when you are demonstrating the Pose/Sequence, and also your execution of the Pose/Sequence.

With your position, mirror your class when you are facing them. What you may want to also consider is to do the demonstration side-on to the class so they can see your profile.

As a large percentage of your class participants will be visual learners, they will mimic what they see you do. Hence, be a clean and precise as possible with your own execution of the Pose/Sequence and any options. And because we are looking to encourage our participants to find their own way with the their Practice, we should come away from physically doing the Practice ourselves, as they will end up copying what you are doing.

Explaining the Poses

Optimal Blueprint

Look at the outer shape and form of the Pose. The particular shape of the body is what defines and distinguishes one Pose from another, but realise that there is an Optimal Blueprint for our body.

The body has an innate intelligence that seeks harmony and health. So, the various parts of the body will instinctively sense our Optimal Blueprint. However, our body may not have the conditioning to move itself into alignment, and without conscious effort to align our body with the Optimal Blueprint, your muscles may spasm in a futile attempt to pull the bones into proper alignment.

So, we should aim to teach our class participants to sense their body position in relation to the Blueprint. From this Optimal Blueprint, they can then spend time in the Pose to play, sense and feel.

Setting the foundation

In any posture, there is a foundation, or that part of the body that connects to the earth. We exist within a field of gravity, a constant force that exerts a downward force on the body and provides the stability from which to rise up, physically and energetically. Gravity roots the body, providing the resistance that creates strength in muscle tissue. Our focus is to expand from this compressive, condensing force.

Aligning the feet

There are four corners to each foot:

1. The mound of the big toe

2. The back of the inner heel

3. The mound of the little toe

4. The back of the outer heel

Spread and root your toes to the ground. Create the sensation of an outward, upward, corkscrewing action and feel the dome of the centre of your foot.

Aligning the hands

When the hands are part of the foundation, they also must be aligned and connected.

The four corners of the hands are:

1. The mound of the index finger

2. The inner heel of the hand

3. The mound of the little finger

4. The outer heel of the hand

Spread and root the fingers and rim of the palm to the ground. Create the sensation of an outward, upward, corkscrewing action and feel the dome of the centre of the centre of your palm.

When the hands are part of the foundation, the creases of the wrists align with each other and the front plane. If you are facing forward on the mat (as in down dog) the creases of the wrists should be parallel to the front edge of your mat. The hands are generally placed shoulder distance apart.

Aligning the knees

In Mountain Pose, the upper leg bones and lower leg bones are vertical and in line with each other. The knees are not bent or hyper-extended. The four corners of each kneecap are square. The sides of the kneecaps are vertical. In standing postures, the knee tracks directly over the ankle, and not beyond.

Aligning the shoulders

The shoulder girdle (collar bones, upper arm bones, shoulder blades) should be placed so that the shoulder blades set into the back of the body. To achieve this, standing in Mountain Pose, elongate the sides of the torso upwards, lift and roll back the shoulders, relaxing the arms to the sides of the body.

Aligning the head and neck

In the head there is more mass forward of the spinal column than behind it. This is readily apparent if viewed from the side of the body. For many of us, the head is held forward of its anatomically neutral position, creating a shortening and a tightness in the shoulders and neck. To release this habitual tightness and bring the head to a neutral position on top of the spinal column, move the top of the throat (where the neck meets the head) back and slightly up. This can be encouraged by elongating the back of the head upward.

ALIGNMENT STUDY:

MOUNTAIN POSE

DOWNWARD FACING DOG

Use of the Breath

The human body is not self-sustaining. It is highly dependent on the external environment for providing it with substances in order to survive, as well as a catch basin into which it can dispose of its wastes. Respiration serves the biological purpose of taking in oxygen and expelling carbon dioxide. Together with the beating of the heart, breathing is life's most continuous muscular action, sustaining us from birth to death.

Part of the fascination with breathing consists in its dual nature, i.e. as something we do and something that happens to us. It is both a voluntary, conscious, muscular action and an involuntary, unconscious, physiological activity. Whether we are awake or asleep, the continuity of our breathing is made certain by the lower centres of the brain. Conversely, the higher centres of the brain regular the conscious control of our breath for speaking, singing or doing breathing exercises.

Emotion plays a considerable part on breathing, though scientific knowledge of the relationship is unsystematic at present. Yoga teaches that of all the physical effects accompanying emotion, breathing changes the most rapidly.

Breath training is an integral part of voice work for actors and singers, and there are many psychotherapeutic uses of breath. Yoga and Zen have long emphasised breathing as part of their spiritual practices. Most health practices and forms of body work recognise breathing improvement as one of their most important goals, with every school emphasising a different aspect of breathing.

Like a car needs fuel to move, the breath is the fuel for movement of the body. It lifts us out of the state of inertia.

In yoga, the breath is what brings the Poses to life. The breath is where the yoga happens; the union of mind and body. Otherwise, what we do is unconscious movement in space. The breath is the key in unlocking the beauty of the Poses. It gently guides us and helps us decide how deep we drop into each Pose. It opens us up. It allows the restriction in body and mind to soften. It tells us softly to back off. It encourages us to explore the Poses from a different angle.

Here are the My Kind of Yoga™ Principles of Breath:

- The inhalation opens the body; the exhalation closes the body
- Controlling the length of the breath gives us better control of the body
- There are four parts to the breath
- Breathe first, then move
- Locational breathing

Open and Close

Very simply, when we breathe in, we open the body. Likewise, when we breathe out, we close the body. In general, the inhalation energises the system and the exhalation calms the system. It intensifies the sensation of opening the body. It also deepens the experience of a back bend.

The exhalation intensifies the sensation of lengthening the back of the body. It deepens the sensation of closing the body.

Of course there are exceptions to the rule, which mainly applies when someone has a lower back issue. In this instance, we inhale, and then move. This restricts the range of motion and provides the lower back more stability.

Controlling the Breath

The Bhagavad Gita states that, "He who is ever of unrestrained mind, devoid of true understanding, his sense-desires then become uncontrollable like the wild horses of a charioteer." How we put this into practice on the yoga mat is through the breath. When we harness the breath, we begin to reign in the mind.

Most people these days are stressed and are unaware of their breathing pattern. Young children breathe deeply and calmly; unless they are upset, of course. Stressed breathing is rapid, shallow and can be erratic. Calm breath is slow, deep and evenly paced.

What we are looking to achieve with the breath in My Kind of Yoga™ is one that is controlled and long. The slower the breath, the more time you have moving in and out of a Pose, and that cultivates more awareness, a sense of mindfulness. When holding a Pose, a long, controlled breath allows for a deeper experience of the Pose. It lets you know if you are ready to go deeper into a Pose, or that you need to back off. Each day is different, so by listening to the breath, you can prevent yourself from going too far.

We control the breath by tightening the glottis (UJJAYI). We look use this way of controlling this breath at all times during a My Kind of Yoga™ class. So, when you are moving through a Sequence, you can move at your own pace, which allows for even greater awareness and mindfulness.

Four Parts of the Breath

There are four natural parts of the breath:

1. Inhale

2. Pause

3. Exhale

4. Pause

Depending on what our intention is, and what we wish to achieve from our practice, we can choose to use the different parts of the breath to intensify the intention.

The pause after the inhalation means that you are holding your breath. This means it will enhance whatever experience you are seeking to achieve with the inhalation.

The pause after the exhalation results in enhancing the effects of the out-breath. A mild word of caution here, as individuals who are approaching the end of their life span may find this pause uncomfortable. It can bring with it a sense of no breath and hence the end of their life.

Breathe first, then move

Let the breath drive the movement. Feel the breath begin, and then let the movement follow.

Allow the breath to drive the movement. Oftentimes we focus on doing the pose, of getting into the Pose and then breathe. Start your breath first, literally for a second or two, and then move into the Pose. It will seem as if the breath created the movement. Imagine that without breath, no movement will occur.

Locational Breathing

Locational Breathing is about assigning a location (hence locational) focus for each part of the breath; the inhale is associated with the chest and the exhale with the abdomen.

The exhalation is a natural process and occurs during the relaxation phase of the breathing cycle. The respiratory muscles relax and the exhalation happens. The idea here is to make it a conscious activity. Use the muscles of your abdomen to exhale, instead of allowing the natural relaxation of the breathing cycle to happen. There is a degree of awareness to it.

The inhale requires a bit more attention and conscious effort. It is about bringing the inhalation into the chest area, by using the muscles of respiration to expand the chest.

Listen to your Class with Good Observation Skills

Listen with attentiveness and care, with all your energy fields. Leading a class is a two-way conversation. As with any conversation, listen for the responses. Responses from your class will be verbal, but more likely to be non-verbal.

HOW CAN YOU TELL IF THEY ARE ENJOYING THE CLASS, OR NOT?

Counter-Poses

Counter-Poses are used to neutralise the possible negative effects of certain strenuous Poses. Think of the last time you were in a long car journey, or even on a plane. After sitting for an extended period of time (hip and spinal flexion), the first thing you usually want to do when you stand up is to stretch (hip and spinal extension). However, if you have been sitting for 12 hours, you would not stretch for 12 hours to neutralise the effect of sitting for so long. Similarly, Counter-Poses are used to return the body to its normal state and to ensure that no tension is carried into the rest of the session, or the rest of the day.

For any one Pose, there may be various Counter-Poses possible, depending on where tension is felt. E.g. a Counter-Pose for a powerful Seated Forward Bend is a gentle Bridge, a static Lying Twist is countered with dynamic Knees-to-Chest.

- Counter-Poses take the body in the opposite direction to where most tension is felt

- If the main Pose was held, then use gentle movement for the Counter-Pose, and vice-versa

- Counter-Poses should be symmetrical

- Counter-Poses should be performed gently

BRIDGE

LYING TWIST

STANDING FORWARD FOLD

Modification Toolbox

As already mentioned, we are different anatomically and physiologically. For this reason, the Poses and the Practices should be modified to suit the individual. Outwardly, you would take into account their physical ability, fitness levels, any existing injuries, joint issues, diseases, illnesses, etc.

What we should also consider is our physical and mental condition is forever changing. Someone could wake up one morning with a stiff neck and someone else with a pain in their shoulder. Someone may find they are full of energy one afternoon, or feel like they are coming down with something.

In addition, we want to empower our class participants so they are able to adapt the Poses to suit their own needs; so that the Practice feels right for them, at any given time.

With all this in mind, modifying the Poses help keep it interesting and help our participants stay engaged throughout the Practice.

Modification Toolbox

Arm variations
Leg variations
Entry and exit variations

Teaching the Feel

As with life, injuries can occur. Generally, in yoga, most of these injuries happen because of inattention or impatience. We often forget that the Poses embody enormous power, which can cut both ways. Used wisely, the Pose are a time-tested tool for self-transformation and self-understanding. However, used recklessly, without awareness or respect, then the possibility of injury increases considerably.

The Sanskrit term ĀSANA derives from the verb "ĀS", which means "to sit", but also "to be present". The word ĀSANA itself continually reminds us that it is important "to be present" when practicing the Poses, to listen carefully to what our body-mind is telling us or asking from us, moment to moment.

Pain vs Sensation

When participants are first starting out with Yoga practice, the sensations felt are often unfamiliar. With more experience, a differentiation can be made between pain and sensation.

Pain in the form of a sudden, jarring sensation, especially in and around joints should not be ignored. The body is sending a signal that there is a misalignment or disconnection that could be injurious.

Sensations of an intense stretch to muscle can be interpreted as pain, but the sensation is much different. You are in control of the amount of sensation felt, as in a seated forward bend. This sensation is an intrinsic part of practice. Often breathing into the sensation draws the mind back into the body and resistance decreases.

Be Mindful

The term "mindfulness" is bantered around a lot in the mind-body world. There are strong links between mindfulness practice and buddhism; yet, there are many mindful practices in hinduism too.

Mindfulness is a quality of presence that is innate in all human beings. Awareness is a natural and beautiful quality of being human that cannot be limited to one particular tradition or country.

Noticing what your judgments of the word mindfulness are before you delve into the practice more deeply is interesting.

WHAT DOES BEING MINDFUL MEAN TO YOU?

Mindfulness is the quality and power of mind that is aware of what's happening — without judgment and without interference. It is like a mirror that simply reflects whatever comes before it. It serves us in the humblest ways, keeping us connected to brushing our teeth or having a cup of tea. It keeps us connected to the people around us, so that we're not simply rushing by them in the busyness of our lives.

We can start the practice of mindfulness meditation with the simple observation and feeling of each breath. Breathing in, we know we're breathing in; breathing out, we know we're breathing out. It's very simple, although not easy. After just a few breaths, we hop on trains of association, getting lost in plans, memories, judgments and fantasies.

This habit of wandering mind is very strong, even though our reveries are often not pleasant and sometimes not even true. As Mark Twain so aptly put it, "Some of the worst things in my life never happened." So we need to train our minds, coming back again and again to the breath, simply beginning again.

Slowly, though, our minds steady and we begin to experience some space of inner calm and peace. This environment of inner stillness makes possible a deeper investigation of our thoughts and emotions. What is a thought— that strange, ephemeral phenomenon that can so dominate our lives? When we look directly at a thought, we see that it is little more than nothing. Yet when it is unnoticed, it wields tremendous power.

Notice the difference between being lost in a thought and being mindful that we're thinking. Becoming aware of the thought is like waking up from a dream or coming out of a movie theatre after being absorbed in the story. Through mindfulness, we gradually awaken from the movies of our minds.

JOSEPH GOLDSTEIN

So, here is a simple method towards practicing mindfulness:

The ABCs of mindfulness

Awareness

just **Be**

Calm and Centred Choices

However, what we want to bear in mind is that the ultimate aim of Yoga practice, goes beyond mindfulness. What we are looking to encourage our participants develop is moving towards mindlessness.

The Art of My Kind of Yoga™

"Words are singularly the most powerful force available to humanity. We can choose to use this force constructively with words of encouragement, or destructively using words of despair. Words have energy and power with the ability to help, to heal, to hinder, to hurt, to harm, to humiliate and to humble."

YEHUDA BERG

The Power of Words

The words we choose and the manner in which they are delivered needs careful consideration. Words, in themselves, are neutral in meaning. The meaning of a word can be powerfully altered by the volume and the tone of delivery.

Our language should reflect the kind of healthy relationship with which to facilitate with your class participants. Consider the following,

- "Stretch your muscles to the limit." Or, "Invite your muscles to open."

- "Push with the arm to twist the spine further." Or, "Keep the arm stable and as you exhale, feel for the moment when the spine is ready to rotate."

- "Breathe in for four counts." Or, "Allow the breath to enter for four counts."

With our words, we can separate mind and body as there is someone doing something to somebody, or we can encourage the action to originate from the inside. In the second instances, the student is asked to self-reflect, rather than simple obey a command.

Through our use of language, we can cultivate independence within our class participants.

Teaching Vocabulary

Set Up Language

- Active Command language:

    - Instructs class participants to form the shapes of the Poses through direct, clear instructions given in active voice.

    - *Step your feet wide, keep your left foot straight ahead and turn your right foot out 90 degrees. Firm your leg muscles and bend your front knee to a right angle, making your front thigh parallel to the floor. Scoop your tailbone, slide your waistline back and lift your chest.*

- Descriptive language:

    - Describes the Pose and gives verbal cues that are an ongoing description of the Pose and action, but without clear directions and implication that the class participants must actually do the actions themselves.

    - *Your feet are wide. Your left foot is straight ahead and your right foot is turned out 90 degrees. Your muscles are firm and your front thigh is bent to a right angle with the front thigh parallel to the floor. Your tailbone is scooping, your waistline is back and your chest is lifting.*

- Passive Voice language:

    - Instructs class participants on how to do the Pose indirectly, making their body the recipient of the action rather than the agent of the action.

    - *Your feet step wide. Your left foot faces straight ahead and your right foot turns out 90 degrees. Your muscles firm and your front thigh bends to a right angle and becomes parallel to the floor. Your tailbone scoops, your waistline moves back and your chest lifts.*

- Gerund-based language:

    - Uses -ing's instead of active commands.

    - *Stepping your feet wide. Keeping your left foot straight ahead ... turning your right foot out 90 degrees .. firming your muscles ... bending your front thigh to a right angle and taking it down to parallel with the floor ... Scooping your tailbone ... moving your waistline back ... and lifting your chest ...*

- Reflective/Feeling Cues:

    - Instruct your class participants to feel and reflect instead of act and do.

    - *Feel your feet wide underneath you. Feel your left leg straight and your right leg turning out. Feel your legs firm and feel yourself come down to a right angle, parallel with the floor. Feel your tailbone scoop. Feel your waistline move back. Feel the lift of your chest.*

    - These cues are very useful when paired with active commands given in an active voice, e.g. "Lift your chest and feel how much deeper your breath is." "Spread your feet into the ground and feel how steady you've become."

TRIANGLE POSE:

BRIDGE POSE:

Developing the Pose

These cues create greater awareness and continuity within a Pose, as well as between Poses.

There are 3 ways to practice linking:

1. **Linking cues within** a Pose. This connects the major parts of the body and major actions within the Pose to the whole Pose, so there is integration of mind, body and awareness. Key words are KEEPING THAT, MAINTAINING ..... DO ...., WITHOUT LOSING THE ...., NOW DO .....

   Press your big toe down as you turn your top thigh out.

   Lift your chest. Keeping that, move your arm back.

2. Giving **direction to actions** with a Pose. Here, you name the place from which the action originates and the place to which the action is going. This form of linking helps integrate mind and body. Key words are FROM and TO.

   Stretch your inner knee to your inner heel.

   Stretch from your hips to your heart to your hands.

3. **Connecting shapes and actions** of one Pose to the next. These cues are external and help teach continuity between Poses, and builds confidence in your class participants through repetitive practice of familiar shapes and actions. Key words are AS THOUGH YOU ARE DOING ..., JUST LIKE YOU DID ..., KEEP THE .... ACTION.

   Strengthen your leg muscles, just like you did in Mountain Pose.

   Keep the feeling of pressing your arms back, just like you did when you were lying on the floor.

LINKING CUES WITHIN WARRIOR 2:

DIRECTION TO ACTIONS WITH THREE-LEGGED DOG:

CONNECTING SHAPES AND ACTIONS OF PLANK AND MOUNTAIN POSE:

Reflective Cues

Reflective cues ask the class participant to reflect on the work they are doing within a Pose. After giving an active cues which tells them to do something, ask them to FEEL, NOTICE, to reflect on the outcome of the action they have just done.

Lift your chest until you feel yourself grow lighter.

Root your legs to the ground and feel how steady you are.

Tuck your tailbone under and lift your lower belly up. Notice the support through your lower back.

Compare the above with giving reflective cues only, or actions that are given with reflective cues:

Feel your chest lifting.

Feel your legs root into the ground.

Feel your tailbone scoop and your lower belly lift.

gently	quietly	being still
being calm	being real	authenticity
with integrity	with honesty	with awareness
energise	dispel	settle
peacefully	effortlessly	easily
blissfully	bind	respond
receive	allow	support
with feeling	appreciately	powerfully
enthusiastically	simply	gratefully
quieten	hover	listen
advance	fold	patiently

Even More Cues

Literal:

Stretch your arms over your head. Reach towards the ceiling with straight arms.

Lift your lower belly up from your pubic bone toward your navel.

Step your feet to the distance of your outer hips.

Biomechanical:

Elevate your shoulders by shrugging them slightly.

Isometrically draw your legs together until your adductors tone.

Maintain the tone in your bicep as you straighten your arm.

Metaphoric:

Open your heart.

Blossom your buttocks.

Melt.

Jargon-based:

Inner spiral your legs.

Use your bandhas.

Do more kidney loop.

Attitudinal:

Offer your heart forwards.

Surrender

Stand strong.

Energetic:

Soften your face.

Lift your kidneys up.

Pull energy up from your feet to your hips.

Assisting

The main intention for adjusting a participant's alignment is to help them feel the Pose more. A Pose is never truly wrong. You are not there to "fix" or correct anything per se. Find what is good in the execution of the Pose and help your participant improve on that.

Make some sort of contact with each participant sometime during the class so they know you are aware of them and you are checking in on them. This could be eye contact, speaking with them, gesture, touch.

Here are some things to consider:

- Take time to observe and decide if you want to adjust at all.

- Could you offer Verbal Adjustments first?

- Look for the most significant misalignments and adjust those first, rather than peripheral parts of inconsequential misalignments.

- Share the love! Avoid spending too much time with any one participant.

Verbal Adjustments

- Use verbal adjustments first. Oftentimes, participants will receive and implement verbal adjustments more readily and quickly than physical adjustments. When they make the adjustments themselves, it increases their awareness and empowers them.

- Offer the verbal adjustments to the whole class in order to bring all your participants to the same level of alignment and action.

- Get to know your participants, so where appropriate, use their name before giving instructions.

- Lower your voice to give individualised and personal instructions or comments to one participants whenever possible.

Hands-on Assistance

- Make sure the participant knows that you will be physically adjusting.

- If making a physical adjustment, carry it out with confidence and without hesitation.

- Place yourself in a position that will give the most effective and beneficial physical adjustment, e.g. make all strong adjustments to standing poses from behind.

- Stabilise your participant with your body or a prop before physically adjusting. Ensure that the foundation is grounded.

- To effectively stretch, the muscle has to be relaxed. Prompt your participant to let go of inappropriately contracted muscles, whilst maintaining the integrity of the Pose.

- Maintain a smooth and steady breath whilst adjusting and you will approach the adjustment with awareness, focus and sensitivity. Also, when you are breathing well, your participant's breath will automatically start to tune into yours, so their breath becomes smooth and steady.

- Be gentle. Be kind.

Types of Adjustments

1. Passive: This is where you are doing all the work. It allows your participant to let go of tensions and move deeper into the position. Your participant will be able to see how far they can go and what is possible, and with time, will learn which muscles to engage and which ones to relax in order to achieve the same position.

2. Active: Both you and your participant are doing the work together. This type of adjustment gives your participant the opportunity to experience how to work specific areas in the Pose.

3. Resistance: This is where you provide resistance to a particular body part. Your participant will have to push against this resistance.

HAVE A GO AT ASSISTING THE FOLLOWING POSES AND MAKE SOME NOTES:

DOWNWARD-FACING DOG

WARRIOR 2

SEATED FORWARD FOLD

STANDING FORWARD FOLD

INTENSE POSE

SEATED BUTTERFLY

Using Your Voice

The Yoga Voice is that slightly monotonous, throaty tone three degrees above a whisper. It can be soothing and effective at creating a gentle environment for yoga, however, it can make the yoga teacher sound like a space cadet and can be mildly irritating to everyone in the class.

From a Chakra perspective, the voice manifests through the throat chakra, which opens with ease and clarity when the body is grounded, the creative juices flowing, the wilful centre strong yet supple, the heart open and the mind clear. How you speak as a teacher reflects where you are in your life, skills and knowledge.

Authenticity is key to engaging your class participants. Let your passion and personality shine through. When you try to sound like a "Yoga Teacher", you'll sound like you're trying to sound like someone you are not, and you could lose sight of what you actually sound like.

Know your audience. Know their skill level. Know the individual's challenges and limitations. Identify the average and offer variations in each. It is as important to understand your audience as it is for the audience to understand you.

Speak in **YOUR yoga voice** and not THE yoga voice. It is possible to be powerfully gentle, just like it is possible to be gently powerful.

There is no need to make unnecessary puns, drop F-bombs, or get heavy-handed with Sanskrit terminology or chanting unless you are willing to own whatever comes from it. There is a fine between arrogance and confidence. That line is called "**having a clue**." You might not be able to tell, but your students always will.

Good teaching is a **dialogue**, not a monologue. Listen and hear what your class participants have to say. Be open to their feedback. Listen to their questions, look for non-verbal cues to help guide the teaching conversation. Teachers skilled at inspiring creation make suggestions based on experience and offer directions with intention.

Be clear on how you wish to be heard before you start speaking. Don't try to sound like someone else. If there is another teacher you admire, establish what their desirable qualities are and work those into your own delivery.

4 Self-Reflect on your Teaching

This is so important, as we strive to continually grow and learn from what we do. Getting feedback from someone you trust helps you with your self-reflection. Keep a Teaching Journal that includes your Lesson Plan, notes from each class or particular students, and self reflect.

WHAT MAY YOU CONSIDER AND REFLECT UPON AFTER YOUR CLASS?

The Role of the Catalyst

WHAT IS A YOGA TEACHER?

HOW DO YOU SEE YOUR ROLE AS A MY KIND OF YOGA™ TEACHER?

The Service of Teaching Yoga

The difference between being a good instructor and a great teacher is authenticity. Instructors pass on skill; teachers share and inspire knowledge. Teaching yoga is great service you can give, and it will change your life.

People come to yoga for many reasons. For many, it is an opportunity to relax and reduce the stress they experience in their lives, and get more supple, and these are the main intentions we hold with My Kind of Yoga™ classes.

Our role as a My Kind of Yoga™ Teacher is to provide inspired support and informed guidance to the people in our classes. Our aim to create safe and nurturing classes where our students can explore, explore and and experience their bodies. New sensations arise in the body. Breathing become a whole new experience and becomes a profound tool of awareness. They will feel better, more vibrant and more alive.

In order to fully serve our students, we should continue to cultivate our own personal practice. With our personal practice, there are two sources of guidance; the outer teacher and the inner teacher. Both listen, watch and use what is necessary to adjust and refine in oder to create a more beautiful experience. The inner teacher is ultimately the best guide. So, allow yourself to fully listen with your physical senses, emotional states and knowledge to find what is right. Sometimes though, we are too close to the issue and it takes a trained, out eye to see and sense what is happening, and so the outer teacher is able to guide the student deeper into their own practice.

In order to be a well-rounded My Kind of Yoga™ Teacher, we need a solid foundation in the following areas:

- **The Science of My Kind of Yoga™** where we understand how the body functions mechanically, modification of the Poses, use of the breath and sequencing of the Poses.

- **The Art of My Kind of Yoga™** which is our teaching skills, which include our voice, verbal instructions, observation skills, demonstration skills, adjustments and our presence.

- **The Business of My Kind of Yoga™** which is how you run your My Kind of Yoga™ business; earn a living whilst upholding the essence of My Kind of Yoga™

- **Living My Kind of Yoga™** which is how we choose to live with the world and its inhabitants

The Business of My Kind of Yoga™
Where You Are Right Now

HOW MUCH ARE YOU CURRENTLY MAKING PER MONTH?

HOW DOES THIS BREAK DOWN FINANCIALLY PER MONTH? E.G.

KINGS WESSEX LEISURE, 5 HOURS X £30 = £600

WHAT ARE YOUR OUTGOINGS EACH MONTH?

Where You Would Like To Be

What would you ideal, perfect average day look like? "Where would you live, what would you house look like, what would you drive, what time would you wake up, what would you do in the morning, what would you have for breakfast, what would you spend the first part of your day doing, what would you have for lunch, who would you want to eat with, what would your friends be like, what would you do for personal fulfilment, what life purpose would you strive towards, what would your business be, what time would you start work, what would you do at work, what would your clients belike to spend time with, what hours would you work, what is your relationship like, what would you do for family time, what would you have for dinner, where would you eat, who would you eat with, what would you do at night, what would your thoughts be as you went to sleep?" - Frank Kern

How much do you CHOOSE to make per month?

What are your various sources of income?

How does this break down financially per month?

E.G.

    Kings Wessex Leisure, 5 hours x £30 = £600

    My Kind of Yoga™ classes, 60 clients over 4 hours x £40 = £2400

My Kind of Yoga™

The basis of My Kind of Yoga™ is to run classes in the community.

Our ideal client is:

"I've always wanted to get into yoga but find the odd class I've tried in the past too complicated and too spiritual for me. I just want a simple, no fluff, straightforward class."

You are relatively new to yoga, or you've been attending yoga classes sporadically for less than 2 years. You may be a member of a health club but want to attend a yoga class closer to home. You love what you've experienced from yoga in the past and want to spend more time cultivating a regular yoga practice.

You can obviously, take this as a premise to further niche your class offerings.

What are your obstacles?

I don't know enough
I'm not enough
They'll find out I'm a fraud
I don't have the right personality to succeed
I'm a failure
Who would want what I have to offer?
I have nothing to offer
I can't compete
I'm not good at marketing
I don't really need as much money as I think I need
I lack focus
I can't do this
I'm not worth it
Now's not the time
I'll get overwhelmed
I can't have it all
They won't pay for this
I don't have what it takes
Who am I to do this?
There are too many competitors
My target group have no money
I'm too disorganised
I'm not motivated enough
I shouldn't charge for this
People won't pay my full fee
I can't sell myself
I'll never make good money at this business
I don't have money to market
I don't like to sell
I'm already too scattered
I can't possibly charge that much!

Marketing

- Posters, flyers & roadside banner

- Free taster classes

- Local newspaper

- Social media

- Networking

Living My Kind of Yoga™

Your time is limited, so don't waste it living someone else's life. Don't be trapped by dogma – which is living with the results of other people's thinking. Don't let the noise of other's opinions drown out your own inner voice. And most important, have the courage to follow your heart and intuition. They somehow already know what you truly want to become. Everything else is secondary.

STEVE JOBS

There are a ton of books out there on yoga philosophy but hand on heart, majority of them pose as heavy duty reading! Most people coming to yoga, at some point, realise that there is some pretty good stuff in there but they do not exactly know how it applies to their daily lives.

Yoga philosophy takes a while to sink in. Part of my mission is to take the very relevant and usable ideas in yoga philosophy and make them accessible to everyday yogis, who seem overwhelmed with first-world issues, like which flavour lip gloss, or how to spend time and money. By adding these guideposts to your Life Toolkit, you will begin to live with more intention and integrity.

On Relationships

Here are five guiding ethical principles (YAMA) which can improve your relationship with others and yourself.

View them as a sort of compass—a way to orient yourself back to the right direction in life when you have been thrown a curveball. They assist you in living a life filled with dignity.

1. **Be Kind (AHIM̐SĀ).** This is the foundation on which the whole yoga practice is built. Cultivate an attitude of love and compassion toward others—toward everyone—even ourselves. It is asking ourselves before doing something—is this harmful or helpful? Am I doing this out of love, or out of fear? It also helps our relationships by getting us to consider the impact we have on others.

2. **Be Truthful (SATYĀ).** Being truthful with others is essential for good relationships. On a basic level, it is about telling the truth to others whilst remembering to Be Kind. Being truthful with ourselves is just as important. But we are pretty good at fooling ourselves about things we do not want to face. Usually, beneath the denial is an awareness of what is really going on—but a lack of acceptance, and acceptance is a necessary condition for change.

3. **Be Respectful (ASTEYA).** Very simply, do not take what is not yours to take. On a more subtle level, it also has to do with not taking what belongs to others, e.g. their time, attention, control, or dignity. Do you respect people enough to be on time? Can you let someone enjoy the spotlight? Do you need to control situations at the expense of others?

4. **Be Mindful (BRAHMACARYA):** Manage your desires and avoid overindulgence. Seek the middle way, on and off the mat. Whilst you can apply this to many aspects of your life, e.g. Facebook usage, Be Mindful with sensual cravings such as chocolate, wine, sexual intercourse, shopping and even yoga.

5. **Be Content (APARIGRAHĀḤ):** Be satisfied with what you have, rather than constantly accumulating shiny new things you really do not need. Much of the time, our stuff is just a distraction from our real lives. Be happy with your own yoga practice. Rejoice in the good fortune of others and ditch jealousy. Seek to simplify rather than accumulate. Graciously give of yourself and your resources.

Kindness and ethical behaviour are necessary if you want true happiness and peace of mind. If you treat yourself badly, you cannot be happy. If you treat others badly, your relationships suffer.

These five principles help take us away from our usual self-centred mindset and start acting out of love, with consideration for the impact we have on others, and on the world. When we feel good about ourselves and what we do, we can have true peace of mind.

[Refer to Yoga Sutra II.30]

HOW CAN YOU COMMIT TO APPLYING THESE PRINCIPLES ON YOUR MAT?

Stuff Gets in the Way

As we get to know ourselves with greater clarity through yoga practice, we start to see the ways we make ourselves (and others) suffer needlessly, because our Stuff (KLEŚA) keeps getting in the way!

The thing is, this Stuff may be so ingrained that we are not even aware of them and they can be present to various degrees. Most of us seem to bounce from one to the other most of our waking hours.

There are basically five of them: ignorance, egoism, attachment, aversion, and clinging to life.

1. **Ignorance (AVIDYĀ):** Referring to the stages of learning, this is unconscious incompetence; our not knowing the way things really are, and really, this is the root of the other Stuff. Despite our best efforts, our brains are only able to take in a certain amount of information, and this limits the way we experience life. We tend to see things only from our own limited perspective.

2. **Egoism (ASMITĀ):** The ego makes decisions on your behalf, often without considering others or the long term consequences. And it has preferences. Oh, how it has preferences! Things we cannot seem to live without and things we cannot stand.

3. **Attachment (RĀGA):** When something brings us pleasure our brains want to repeat that experience and on some basic level we expect the things (and people) that give us a moment's pleasure to make us happy. I'm pretty sure life wouldn't end if I couldn't have my iPhone, but I hate to think about it. I'm attached to about a million other things; we all are. Even though we know that looking for happiness outside ourselves doesn't work, it does not stop us from acting as if it did, to the point that we do not even question our desires.

4. **Aversion (DVEṢA):** We let our attachment to having things the way we want them, to having our preferences catered to get in the way of our happiness. When we are confronted with something we do not like or did not want, somehow it becomes much more than that. The one little thing that can put you in a bad mood. Your football team loses. You show up for your favourite yoga class only to find out there is a substitute teacher (oh, the horror!). What if we could just coexist with the things (and people) we do not like, without getting upset about it?

5. **Clinging to life (ABHINIVEŚĀḤ):** Or simply, fear of death. Many psychologists and philosophers believe that this is the one thing we all have in common – whether people admit it, or are aware of it or not. It can take the form of a midlife crisis, extreme religiosity, fear of the unknown, or almost any flavour of neurosis out there. This one goes pretty deep.

[Refer to Yoga Sutra II.3]

So what can you do when Stuff arises? Here is a simple recipe is to follow:

The 4 A's: Attention, Acknowledge, Allow, Accept

Pay **Attention** to what arises in your mind. Try to notice when one of the Stuff comes up.

Acknowledge what comes up. Do not try to deny or push it away. If you are craving a Ben & Jerry's whilst on your yoga mat, admit it to yourself! By being aware, you can deal with it.

Allow the Stuff to come, and to go. Imagine your mind has an in-door and an out-door. Keep both doors open and try to let go of the Stuff rather than fight or give in to them.

Accept. This Stuff is part of being human. It is not so much to be free from them (though that would be nice) as to learn to coexist with them and not let them control or define you.

On Personal Practice

This is where my wish for My Kind of Yoga™ comes to the forefront. By cultivating good, personal habits toward ourselves that serve us, we live better lives.

The practice of yoga is simple and is summed up in the Yoga Sutra (II.1) in three steps:

The Practice of Yoga

Commit (TAPAḤ)

Reflect (SVĀDHYĀYA)

Surrender (ĪŚVARAPRAṆIDHĀNANI)

Like a recipe, mix the Personal Practice ingredients on your yoga mat consistently, with full effort, over a long period of time. Season liberally with kindness as needed. Remember it is perfectly normal to overcook and have it spill off your yoga mat. Just be mindful and turn down the heat.

Rinse and repeat.

Our lives are infinitely complicated, we are all different, and we cannot make sweeping generalisations about how change happens.

That said, the process of Kriya Yoga that Patanjali describes in the Yoga Sutras (II.1) is an amazingly concise recipe for removing the obstacles that stand in the way of us being our best selves. And that is what the process of transformation in yoga is really about. It is not about making you someone you are not. It is about uncovering all the junk, gunk, and conditioning that have warped and obscured your best, authentic, true Self.

You do not have to do anything special, or do any particular type of yoga, but you do have to practice consistently and wholeheartedly. Be enthusiastic with your practice. The word comes from the Greek word, 'entheos', meaning 'from God'. And, at some point, subtle but positive changes start to occur in your life off the mat.

In a nutshell, the Practice of Yoga encourages us to: show up and do the work, continue to seek out and be open to new information, and let go of the outcome.

Commit

We all have days in which we do not want to go to work, exercise or do something that is good for us. We may want to stay in bed all day, or eat the entire box of chocolates, rather than get up and draw open the curtains.

So, what can help us work through our resistance? Commitment.

We need to learn how to endure the healthy discomfort of change. Just as we learn to stay calm and centred through discomfort on the mat, we learn to observe our resistance off the mat. Sometimes emotional discomfort is an indication that something in our life is destructive and needs to change. Or it can be a pattern we are stuck in, fuelled by negative, self-defeating thoughts. Other times, it's just what happens when we try something new and get out our comfort zone. Either way, we habitually tend to avoid things that make us uncomfortable, reaching for the first thing that alleviates our discomfort, be it alcohol, sex, or food. Learn to pay attention to the discomfort in life. Learn to listen, endure and learn from it, rather than trying to avoid or medicate it away.

Being committed is an act of kindness. It is learning to stay present and connected to our own kindness even when things are difficult. There are going to be times in all of our lives when we are uncomfortable, or worse. The best we can do is to use these times to learn and become better versions of ourselves.

So, remind yourself of the big picture, why you are and should do something, why it is good for you. To get the benefits of any practice, we need sustained effort and discipline over time; to remain committed to the cause, to your 'why'.

Let go of the internal chatter and just focus on doing what you know you really need to do. Just by showing up, you have already made progress. You have strengthened your commitment. One little change every day adds up to a lot of progress – and momentum – before too long.

Reflect

Learning and study are vital to personal development. Whether we are practicing a new hobby, studying the yoga sutras or a new language, learning is good for your brain and your mental health.

In addition, we should regularly engage in honest self-reflection, which should include examining not only the things we could improve, but the things we have done well too. Looking in the mirror honestly and kindly, with our commitment in mind, we can begin to see where we need to make changes in the direction of becoming the person we want to be.

We have all struggled with a Yoga Pose before. You just do not get it, it does not feel good, and then one day you get an amazing adjustment from a skilled teacher and you get it. It took something or someone outside yourself to get you there, and you had to be ready to receive it.

Whilst we can get guidance of books and teachers in our study of yoga off the mat, for it to be transformative, we have to be willing to apply it to ourselves. We have to be willing to change the way we think and do things, which might mean giving something up or admitting we were wrong about something.

Surrender

Admittedly, a certain amount of control of ourselves is desirable. However, as much as we would like to be in control of our lives, at some point, we have to acknowledge and admit that we cannot control everything.

Let go of the way you view the world and open up to something different, something beyond the confines of your limited worldview. Let go of your own ego and lead your life in the service of higher principles. The world does not exist for your convenience. It is about reminding yourself, constantly: it is not about you.

Let go of having to control everything, including the outcome. All you can really do is make an honest, non-selfish effort toward doing the right thing. That is all you can control, and all you need to be concerned with.

Show up, do your best, stay open to new information, and when it's all said and done, let it go. Be less concerned with getting somewhere than sticking with this basic process, and shift will happen.

Remember, it is not about you and the ultimate outcome is not totally up to you.

How can you apply this to you as a Teacher?

The My Kind of Yoga™ Teacher Tribe

Now that you are part of the My Kind of Yoga™ Teacher Tribe, we see you as part of our family. We will grow, learn and support each other, as we travel lightly along the Yoga path.

It is not a coincidence that you are here on this journey. I believe there is a greater design to our life's work and our purpose in this lifetime. So whether you understand what you are all about, or whether you have no idea where you are going, trust in the process. TAPAS, SVADHYAYA and ISVARA PRANIDHANA … discipline, self study and surrender to grace.

This journey is transformational; for you, for us and for those you meet along the way. You have the potential to touch hearts and lives, as long as you lead with a soft heart. In order to do that, you will have to start living on, and off your mat.

We would obviously love to keep sharing space and ideas with you so that we touch even more lives with yoga. With that in mind, you can always reach out to us to become an Ambassador.

WHAT CAN YOU PERSONALLY DO TO START LIVING ON, AND OFF YOUR MAT?

MAKE A COMMITMENT TO YOURSELF

WHAT WILL YOU DO TO SEE IT THROUGH?

In Closing
My Wish For You

You are capable of more than you realise. With some effort, patience, and willingness, you will exceed your own expectations in practice. It will take time to build the strength and/or flexibility that a lot of poses require, but your mind state is just as important. Quieten the voice in your head that tells you that you will never be able to do that. Stay open and stay committed.

You can learn to relax. The ability to relax is a skill that takes time to develop. Yoga helps, breathing exercises help, meditation helps, working with your self-talk helps. Stick with it. Just because you didn't relax today in Corpse Pose or yesterday at the traffic jam, does not mean you cannot.

Ditch trying to be perfect. There is no one right way to do a pose, and no finish line. If you ask ten different yoga teachers about a point of alignment, you may get ten different answers. Listen to what everyone has to say, and find what works best for your body.

Practice, practice, practice. You will get a lot more out of your practice if you practice at least three times a week; even more if you practice everyday. Consistency is the mother of mastery.

There is a time for everything. There is a time to push forwards, and there is a time to pull back. Practice a lot and challenge yourself, but also give yourself plenty of time to rest. Do a My Kind of Yoga™ GROUNDED at least once a week. Do not feel guilty about taking a day off. Your body and mind will thank you.

There is no 'bad' practice. It does not matter if you could not get into that arm balance today. Do not feel bad if your heart was not in your practice one day. It is what it is. Maybe you can reflect on what was going on and learn something from it, or maybe not. Remember, it is showing up that counts.

Remember to be kind to yourself. We bring all of our personality traits to the mat so if you tend to be self-critical or perfectionistic, it will show up in your practice. If you find this a challenge, ask yourself how you might encourage a good friend or child in their practice. Extend that same sort of encouragement and kindness to yourself.

When you come to class, you are supporting your community. Your presence, your efforts and your practice support the others in the class, and enhance their practice. You may not realise that you inspire someone, or that they enjoy your presence in class.

I am a student too, and I am constantly learning, working through my thoughts and reflections on and off my mat. I do not know it all. I cannot do all the big poses either. I fight my own battles, just like you. I am just fortunate to be able to share what I learn with you, and I hope it is helpful.

I appreciate you. I know you did not have to come here, and I am happy and thankful when you do. I also learn from you. I am inspired by you. I appreciate your feedback. You make me a better teacher.

What is also true is that yoga is not about feeling good all the time. Yes, we can love the kick from yoga when we start feeling the benefits, but as transformative as yoga is, it's not going to get rid of all your bad feelings and problems. Yoga can cultivate a clarity that brings painful, unacceptable things about your life into focus so that sometimes things get worse before they get better.

Forget about trying to rid yourself completely of sadness, anger and fear. These emotions are not the problem. They are a gift that protect and help you stay on track. The real problem is that we try to deny, run from or cover up these feelings and end up making things worse in the process.

Know that your "stuff" - the self-doubt, criticism, intimidation, judgment or whatever your drag onto your mat - is just that, stuff. They are not fact, not truth. With increased awareness comes the ability to see your stuff for what it is, and to not get caught up in it.

Your mat is like a portable laboratory where you can try new ways of being, doing, and relating to yourself. It is allows us the opportunity to create habits that serve us. It affords us the opportunity to step out of our usual, autopilot way of going through life. You get to practice being aware, and kind, and catch yourself with a negative thought process and choose a different thought.

Sometimes less is more. I know you want to get stronger and I appreciate your hard work and dedication. But when you climb out on that limb and go to a place in a pose in which you cannot breathe or maintain calm, you are risking your safety. Often when we pull back just slightly, we can actually work harder, better, and get stronger.

Always remember that the Poses should serve you, not the other way around. They should feel yummy, and not yucky. The Pose is there to make you healthier, to wake you up, to help prepare your body and mind for something more important off the mat. If your practice is serving the pose, you are practicing ego yoga.

The breath really is important. Breathing mindfully helps focus the mind, it calms the nervous system, makes you more aware, and can keep you from getting hurt.

Finally, know that none of us, especially me, remembers this stuff all the time. We all have crazy days, full of self-doubt, unable to focus on the breath or anything else for that matter. You are not alone. No one said we have to be perfect on this path.

I am where I am today because of you. It excites me to watch you progress, and I am blessed to be part of your practice. I value our relationship; it makes me a better teacher.

I wish you all of the above, and when you can take your yoga off your mat to the difficult, messy parts of your life, you are really doing yoga.

Follow you joy …

Journeying Within

By Ann Jensen

Slow and steady, please do not force

Always do your best, of course

Stay within your comfort zone

Following your breath alone

Daily practice is the key

And with a touch of levity

Oh, dear friend, it won't be long

Until you're flexible and strong

Energise from head to feet

To generate internal heat

Enjoy the beauty that you see

And gaze into infinity

As you quiet down you'll find

You'll be blessed with peace of mind

But cultivate your highest goal

The perfect stillness of your soul

Appendices

Understand the Poses

Deciding on the appropriate Lesson Plan assumes an understanding of the Poses.

Over the years, the yoga world has adapted and drawn from other disciplines so that there are now a huge range of poses available; some are not in the older yoga texts.

Some transitional moves have been adapted now into Poses in their own right. Other Poses probably do not even have a Sanskrit name!

With My Kind of Yoga™, we want to make yoga practice accessible to the masses; we want to keep it simple and drop the fluff. Hence, we will use English terminology for the Poses, rather than use Sanskrit. If you are interested in the Sanskrit terms (this can be useful when you are exploring the Poses in more depth and trawl the internet or more traditional texts), then a list is located the back of this manual.

The Poses can be classified dependent on their function, and in My Kind of Yoga™, we classify them as follows:

- Standing

- Balances

- Back Bends

- Forward Bends

- Hip Openers

- Twists

- Inversions

- Restoratives

Standing Poses

These Poses are essential for developing body awareness, muscular strength (especially in the legs) and balance. The entire body is affected strongly by the force of gravity and therefore has to work strenuously. Standing Poses encourage circulation as well as a balanced flow of energy through the body.

Balance Poses

Aside from the obvious of improving balance, Balance Poses also bring a sense of being centred and focused. You have to centre the mind in order to balance well. Arm Balance Poses require courage, strength, and stamina, and are perhaps the most exhilarating class of postures.

Back Bend Poses

Backbends open the front of the body. Gravity and habitual closure of the front body due to posture can round the back and close off the front body, both physically and emotionally. They invigorate the nervous system and can help to release held emotions. As these postures enliven the nervous system, time of day should be considered for intense backbend practice as they can create insomnia if practiced too late in the evening.

Forward Bend Poses

These Poses stretch the back of the body, closing the front where our organs of perception are oriented. Compared to Backbends, the effects here are generally more introverted, soothing, and calming to the nervous system. In order for a forward bend to have a beneficial effect, the lower back should be slightly concave and the spine extended, tipping the pelvis forward, before folding the torso forward. It may be necessary to sit on a block or blanket to achieve this. If standing, keep legs firm and simply fold partway, with hands supported on legs.

Twisting Poses

Twists are very functional in maintaining a supple spine. They also give the internal organs a massage and are both somewhat invigorating and balancing to the nervous system. To be of most benefit, one part of the twist must stay stable while the other part moves. The most mobile part of the spine, the neck, will often unconsciously move before the less mobile parts of the spine. Move the torso, both left and right sides equally, into a twist and allow the chest to initiate the depth of the posture. Keep a firm foundation throughout the twist.

Inverted Poses

Being upside down literally changes your point of view. Inversions encourage circulation by allowing gravity to reverse the flow of blood. There is generally some fear connected to being upside down since it is disorienting initially. Be patient and move slowly.

Hip Opening Poses

Hip openers can release lower back pain and misalignment in the legs. Because of our preference for sitting in chairs, the muscles and connective tissue of the hips tighten over time and limit range of motion. This coupled with weak abdominal muscles creates a situation where it becomes difficult for many adults even to sit comfortably on the ground. In order for the front and back of the hips to open, a balance of strengthening and flexibility is key. Also, the bone structure in the pelvic area can vary greatly from person to person, allowing some great freedom of movement and others restriction.

Restorative Poses

These postures are by nature designed to relax and restore energy. Corpse Pose is the ultimate restorative posture, in which the challenge is allowing true relaxation—a release of muscular tension and of controlled breath while remaining conscious. The body has an innate ability to heal itself. Restorative postures allow a greater flow of energy in the areas targeted. Because of the total relaxation needed, restorative postures should be primarily supine and possibly supported by props.

Sun Salutation

"With hands in prayer I face the sun, feeling love and joy in my heart. I reach out and let the sun fill me with warmth. I bow before the sun's radiance and place my face to the ground in humble respect. I lift my face to the sun and then remember, to achieve such heights, I must be as the dust of the earth. I stretch up towards its light trying to reach the greatest heights and again surrender. I stand tall as I remember the true sun is within me."

Samskrti & Veda, 1985

SURYA = sun; NAMASKĀR = salutations

The original Sun Salutations was not a sequence of postures, but rather a sequence of sacred words. The Vedic tradition, which predates classical yoga by several thousands of years, honoured the sun as a symbol of the Divine. Vedic mantras to honour the sun were traditionally chanted at sunrise. The full practice includes 132 passages and takes more than an hour to recite. After each passage, the practitioner performs a full prostration, laying his body face-down on the ground in the direction of the sun in an expression of devotion.

The Sun Salutations is a series of 12 dynamic Poses described in contemporary manuals of Hatha Yoga. However, the origins of Sun Salutations in modern Hatha Yoga are more mysterious as there is no reference to ĀSANA as 'Sun Salutation' in traditional yoga texts.

It can be said that the Sun Salutations is composed of three elements: form, energy and rhythm. The 12 Poses are said to generate Prāna. Their performance, in a steady, rhythmic sequence, reflects the rhythms of the universe; the 24-hours of the day, the 12 zodiac phases of the year and the biorhythms of the body. The application of this form and rhythm to the body-mind complex generates the transforming force which produces a fuller and more dynamic life.

The traditional 12 Poses are:

1. Mountain

2. Extended Mountain

3. Standing Forward Fold

4. Lunge

5. Plank

6. Eight-Point

7. Upward-facing Dog

8. Downward-facing Dog

9. Lunge

10. Standing Forward Fold

11. Extended Mountain

12. Mountain

My Kind of Yoga™ Sun Salutation

The Sun Salutation that we tend to use in My Kind of Yoga™ has been adapted from the one used in Astanga Vinyasa Yoga.

We offer modifications with the transitions to make it more accessible to each individual.

1. Mountain

2. Extended Mountain

3. Standing Forward Fold

4. [Step or jump back to ...] Plank

5. Crocodile

6. Upward-facing Dog

7. Downward-facing Dog

8. [Step or jump forwards to ...]

9. Standing Forward Fold

10. Extended Mountain

11. Mountain

Key My Kind of Yoga™ Poses

Bird	BAKĀSANA
Bridge	DWI PADA PITHAM
Butterfly (seated and lying)	BHADRĀSANA
Cat (upward-facing and downward-facing)	MARJARYĀSANA
Child's (and twisted)	BALĀSANA
Cobra	BHUJANGĀSANA
Corpse	ŚAVĀSANA
Crocodile	CATURĀṄGA DAṆDĀSANA
Downward-Facing Dog	ADHO MUKHA SVANĀSANA
Easy Sitting	SUKHĀSANA
Extended Side Angle (Extended Warrior 2)	UTTHITA PĀRŚVA KOṆĀSANA
Fire Log (Modified Half Lotus)	AGNITAMBHĀSANA
Forward Fold variations	PAŚCIMATĀNĀSANA / UTTĀNĀSANA
Garland (Hindi Squat)	MĀLĀSANA
Glute Stretch (seated and lying)	n/a
Intense Pose (full and half)	UTKATĀSANA / ARDHA UTKATĀSANA
Knees-to-Chest	ĀPANĀSANA
Locust	ŚALABHĀSANA
Lunge (high, low, wide, kneeling)	AŚWA SANCHALANĀSANA
Lying Twist	JATHARA PARIVṚTTI
Mountain	TADĀSANA
Plank	UTTHITA CATURĀṄGA DAṆDĀSANA
Side Plank	VASIṢTHĀSANA
Swan Pose + variations	EKA PĀDA RĀJAKAPOTĀSANA
Upward-Facing Dog	ŪRDHVA MUKHA SVANĀSANA
Warrior 2	VIRABHADRĀSANA 2

Models

As Yoga is such an ancient approach to the body, life and living, it makes sense that there are different models, ways of looking at the human body and how it works. Some models include:

- Functional Web

- Ayurvedic constitution [DOSHA]

- Mind states [GUNA]

- Energy [PRANA]

- Channels of Energy [NADI] and CHAKRA

- Subtle Bodies [KOSHA]

Having a grasp of models like these can help give you guidance on what Intention to use with your classes.

Functional Web

There are three holistic networks that make up the human body; the neural net, the fluid net and the fibrous net.

Myofascial lines are interconnected strands of fascia and muscle bundles. The fascia not only provides an important structural function, but is involved in communication, wound healing and immune function. Fascia interpenetrates and surrounds muscles, bones, organs, nerves, blood vessels and other structures. The myofascial net is an uninterrupted, three-dimensional web of connective tissue and muscles that extends from head to toe, from front to back, from interior to exterior.

As the fascia envelopes the entire body, any workout would ultimately affect the body as a whole. This is the reason why it is beneficial to use whole, integrated body movements to improve fascial health. Force is equally distributed through the whole system, thereby easing joint tensions.

Here are some insights into training the neuromyofascial web:

1. Use variation, rather than a repetitive program better for a smooth fascia.

2. Whole body movements by engaging long myofascial chains

3. Adaptive movement. Avoid working with upper level loads all the time.

For the purposes of My Kind of Yoga™, there are 3 that we want to bear in mind:

1) Superficial Back Line. The plantar fascia is connected to the erector spinae and skull. From toes to nose. From an applied functional perspective, the superficial back line actively holds the body in an erect position when standing. In strengthening backbend postures like Locust Pose, the superficial back line is activated anti-gravity and strengthened. In forward bending postures, like Standing Forward Bend, the superficial back line is stretched.

2) Superficial Front Line. The anterior tibialis is connected to the sternocleidomastoid. From toes to nose. The Superficial Front Line (SFL) acts to contract the front of the body. A perfect example of this is Boat Pose. In this pose the entire SFL is anti-gravity. The Superficial Front Line stretches in backbends and one of the quintessential backbends is Camel Pose. The SFL is being lengthened in this pose.

3) Lateral Line. The Lateral Line brackets each side of the body from the medial and lateral mid-point of the foot around the outside of the ankle and up the lateral aspect of the leg and thigh, passing along the trunk in a 'basket weave' or shoelace pattern under the shoulder to the skull in the region of the ear.

WHICH POSE WOULD STRENGTHEN THE LATERAL LINE?

WHICH POSE WOULD STRETCH THE LATERAL LINE?

Ayurvedic Constitution (DOSHA)

Ayurveda is an ancient health care tradition that has been practiced in India for at least 5,000 years. The word comes from the Sanskrit terms AYUR (life) and VEDA (knowledge).

Though Ayurveda, or Ayurvedic medicine, was documented in the sacred historical texts known as the Vedas many centuries ago, Ayurveda has evolved over the years and is now integrated with other traditional practices, including yoga.

Health care is a highly individualised practice under Ayurvedic principles, which state that everyone has a specific constitution, or PRAKRUTI, that determines his or her physical, physiologic and mental character and disease vulnerability.

PRAKRUTI is determined by three "bodily energies" called DOSHA, of which there are three basic dosha, and though everyone has some features of each, most people have one or two that predominate. Thought to be condensed from different combinations of the primal elements earth, water, fire, air, and ether, the DOSHA are the life energies behind all of our bodily functions. Each one commands a specific force in the body and is associated with certain sensory qualities.

PITTA energy is linked to fire, and is thought to control the digestive and endocrine systems. People with PITTA energy are considered fiery in temperament, intelligent and fast-paced. When PITTA energy is out of balance, ulcers, inflammation, digestive problems, anger, heartburn and arthritis can result.

VATA energy is associated with air and space, and is linked to bodily movement, including breathing and blood circulation. VATA energy is said to predominate in people who are lively, creative, original thinkers. When out-of-balance, VATA types can endure joint pain, constipation, dry skin, anxiety and other ailments.

KAPHA energy, linked to earth and water, is believed to control growth and strength, and is associated with the chest, torso and back. KAPHA types are considered strong and solid in constitution, and generally calm in nature. But obesity, diabetes, sinus problems, insecurity and gallbladder issues can result when KAPHA energy is out of balance, according to Ayurvedic practitioners.

According to Ayurvedic beliefs, factors such as stress, unhealthy diet, weather and strained relationships can all influence the balance that exists between a person's DOSHA. These unbalanced energies in turn could leave individuals more susceptible to disease.

Mind Body Questionnaire, *David Simon (1997)*

Use the scale to indicate how characteristic each statement is of you.
5 = very like you, 4 = moderately, 3 = somewhat, 2 = slightly and 1 = not at all like you.

	1	2	3	4	5
Section 1					
My mind is very active					
I like trying out new ideas and having new experiences					
I get restless if I'm not constantly on the move					
I speak quickly and am a lively conversationalist					
Under stress, I worry or become anxious					
I am a light sleeper					
I am thin or underweight for my height					
My appetite is variable; sometimes I am hungry and other times I have a force myself to eat					
Under stress or when traveling, I am likely to have constipation					
My digestion is frequently irregular with gas or bloating					
My feet and hands are often cold					
My skin is often dry or flaky					
TOTAL for SECTION 1:					
Section 2					
I have a very discriminating mind					
I tend to be compulsive and have difficulty stopping once I've started a project					
I am a perfectionist and am intolerant of errors					
I often feel time pressure and become impatient easily					
When stressed, I become irritable or lose my temper					
I have a strong appetite and can eat large quantities of food if I choose					
I often have indigestion or heartburn					
Under stress, I am more likely to get diarrhoea than constipation					
I feel rested with less than eight hours of sleep					
My hair shows early thinning or greying, or a tendency toward a reddish colour					
I am most comfortable in cooler environments					
My skin is sensitive, sunburns or breaks out easily					
TOTAL for SECTION 2:					

	1	2	3	4	5
Section 3					
I am sweet-natured and forgiving					
I accumulate things: I don't like to let go of things even if I don't expect to use them again					
I have difficulty leaving a relationship, even after it is no longer nourishing					
I am a good listener. I tend to speak only when I feel I have something important to say.					
I am calm by nature and seldom lose my temper					
I deal with conflict by withdrawing					
Once I've learned something, I usually have good retention					
I sleep deeply for eight or more hours each night					
I commonly experience sinus congestion or excessive phlegm, or suffer with asthma					
My skin is usually soft and smooth					
I gain weight easily and have difficulty losing extra pounds					
TOTAL for SECTION 3:					

Results:

VATA
PITTA
KAPHA

Mind States (GUNA)

Alongside the DOSHA, there are also three mind states (GUNA). The predominate GUNA of the mind acts as a lens that effects our perceptions and perspective of the world around us. The three GUNA are TAMAS, RAJAS and SATTVA.

TAMAS is a state of darkness, inertia, inactivity and materiality. It manifests from ignorance and deludes all beings from their truths. To reduce TAMAS, avoid tamasic foods (e.g. heavy meats, and foods that are spoiled, chemically treated, processed or refined), over sleeping, over eating, inactivity, passivity and fearful situations.

RAJAS is a state of energy, action, change and movement. The nature of RAJAS is of attraction, longing and attachment and it strongly binds us to the fruits of our work. To reduce RAJAS, avoid rajasic foods (e.g. fried foods, spicy foods, and stimulants), over exercising, over work, loud music, excessive thinking and consuming excessive material goods.

SATTVA is a state of harmony, balance, joy and intelligence. It is the guna that yogi/nis strive towards as it reduces RAJAS and TAMAS and therefore makes liberation possible. To increase SATTVA, eat sattvic foods (e.g. whole grains and legumes and fresh fruits and vegetables that grow above the ground), and enjoy activities and environments that produce joy and positive thoughts. All of the yogic practices were developed to create SATTVA in the mind and body.

Energetic Body (PRANA)

Through their exploration of the body and breath, the ancient yogis discovered that life force energy (PRANA) could be further subdivided into five VAYU (winds). These all have very subtle yet distinct energetic qualities, including specific functions and directions of flow. These yogis were alleged to be able control and cultivate these VAYU by simply bringing their focus and awareness to them. Through this conscious control and cultivation they were not only able to create optimal health and well-being.

So by cultivating a basic awareness of one or more of the VAYU will help us deepen our awareness of body and breath to enrich our yoga practice. The two most important VAYU are PRANA VAYU and APANA VAYU.

1. PRANA VAYU is situated in the head and its energy pervades the chest region. The flow of PRANA VAYU is inwards and upward. It nourishes the brain and the eyes and governs reception of all things: food, air, senses, and thoughts. It is the fundamental energy in the body, and directs and feeds into the other four. To experience PRANA VAYU: Close your eyes, sit or stand with a long spine and relaxed body, and as you inhale feel an energy flowing up the torso from the belly to the third-eye.

2. APANA VAYU is situated in the pelvic floor and its energy pervades the lower abdomen. Its flow is downwards and out, and its energy nourishes the organs of digestion, reproduction and elimination. It governs the elimination of all substances from the body: carbon monoxide, urine, stool, etc. To experience APANA VAYU: Close your eyes, sit or stand with a long spine and relaxed body, and as you exhale feel an energy flowing down the torso from the top of the head to the tailbone.

3. VYANA VAYU is situated in the heart and lungs and flows throughout the entire body. It moves from the centre of the body to the periphery. It governs circulation of all substances throughout the body, and assists the others with their functions. To experience VYANA VAYU: Close your eyes, sit or stand with a long spine and relaxed body, and as you inhale feel the breath radiating outward from the navel to the arms and legs.

4. UDANA VAYU is situated in the throat and it has a circular flow around the neck and head. It functions to "hold us up" and governs speech, self-expression and growth. <u>To experience UDANA VAYU</u>: Close your eyes, sit or stand with a long spine and relaxed body, and as you inhale and exhale feel the breath circulating around and through the head and neck.

5. SAMANA VAYU is situated in the abdomen with its energy centred in the navel. Its flow moves from the periphery of the body to the centre. It governs the digestion and assimilation of all substances: food, air, experiences, emotions and thoughts. <u>To experience SAMANA VAYU</u>: Close your eyes, sit or stand with a long spine and relaxed body, and as you inhale and exhale feel the breath rising and falling in the front, sides and back of the torso.

APPLICATION

1. PRANA VAYU: Create a focus to lift, lengthen and open the upper body

2. APANA VAYU: Create a focus to ground and stabilise the lower body

3. VYANA VAYU: Create a focus of strength and fluid movement body

4. UDANA VAYU: Create a focus to maintain a long spine and a correct posture

5. SAMANA VAYU: Create a focus to open and relax the body

Channels of Energy (NADI) and CHAKRA

All of us possess a network of nerves and sensory organs that interprets the outside physical world. From a Yoga perspective, within us resides a subtle system of channels (NADI) and centres of energy (CHAKRA) which look after our physical, intellectual, emotional and spiritual being.

The word CHAKRA means "wheel" and very simply, from how I have been taught, yoga is about getting these wheels to spin smoothly so that energy flows well throughout our bodies (KUNDALINI). For most of us, our wheels are clogged up with gunk. Now, I know there are lots of other theories behind the CHAKRA, however, coming from a scientific background, I can appreciate energy flow. I also wonder if each CHAKRA is also a junction of nerves along the spinal chord, and therefore, any disturbance to the junction, communication along the nervous system and therefore the rest of the body is affected.

As a map, each CHAKRA has several spiritual qualities. These qualities are intact within us, and even though they might not always be manifest, they can never be destroyed. When the KUNDALINI is awakened, these qualities start manifesting spontaneously and express themselves in our life.

The many approaches to Yoga practice means that there are various approaches to awaken KUNDALINI, including breath work (PRANAYAMA) and meditation.

From a mystical, esoteric perspective, enlightenment and good health requires the free flow of PRANA (the life force) and the proper balance of all the CHAKRA. When they are all aligned and balanced, it produces a positive energy field. When they are severally out of balance it produces a negative state or charge which produces unwanted results. The three lower chakras serve the bodies physical needs while the other five are associated with the spiritual realm.

From a scientific perspective, the practice of Yoga has shown to decrease blood pressure, lower stress levels and slow the rate of ageing common in the western world. The various poses or postures exercise the entire body; both externally and internally. It helps in the removal of all waste both physical and cellular. It improves muscle tone, protects and repairs joints and ligaments. Yoga helps within the brain by improving focus, balance, discipline, application, and understanding

The Crown CHAKRA means "thousand petalled" and is not, strictly speaking, part of the CHAKRA system. We could see it as the petals unfolding when all the other CHAKRA are flowing freely, and hence, affects your overall aura.

Chakra	Eastern	Western	Symbol
Root [MULADHARA]	Earth Lower limbs	Reproductive organs Helps produce sex hormones	
Sacral [SWADHISTHANA]	Water Sexual energy	Kidneys Enhances drainage of waste from lymphatic system	
Navel [MANIPURA]	Fire Personal power Storage of life force (Prana)	Adrenal glands Controls the over usage of adrenaline	
Heart [ANAHATA]	Air Compassion Love Respect	Heart and lungs Strengthens the circulatory system, lowers blood pressure, improves deep breathing	
Throat [VISHUDDI]	Ether Self expression Energy Endurance	Thyroid gland Helps to secrete less metabolic hormones (slows ageing)	
Brow [AJNA]	Senses Intuition Telepa	Pituitary gland Helps to secrete less stress hormones	
Crown [SAHASRARA]	Intuition Awareness Spirituality	Brain Control centre, signals the body, focus, knowledge	

Understand the Subtle Bodies (KOSHA)

The KOSHA, "layers" or "sheaths," map out our personal landscape, charted by yogic sages some 3,000 years ago. Written about in the UPANISHAD, the KOSHA model navigates an inner journey—starting from the periphery of the body and moving towards the core of the self. While this may sound esoteric, we need to appreciate that there are energetic aspects to our bodies and minds that are subtle and somehow affect us. When teaching, we need to realise that the KOSHA are both a practical and profound contemplative tool that can help deepen yoga practice.

According to the map of the KOSHA, we are composed of five layers, sheaths, or bodies. Like Russian dolls, each metaphorical "body" is contained within the next. As a metaphor, the KOSHA help describe what it feels like to do yoga from the inside; the process of aligning what in contemporary language we often call "mind, body, and spirit".

Physical body	ANNA MAYA	Food and the elements of earth, water and fire Equates with Tamas
Breath or life-force body	PRANA MAYA	Prana or life force Includes Nadis and Chakras
Mental body	MANO MAYA	Elements of air and space Seat of the ego Cognition, perception We have opinion, concept, belief, viewpoint
Wisdom body	VIJNANA MAYA	Beyond individuation Insight and discrimination from a cosmic view Touching into the psychic realms Deeper recognition of the unity of all consciousness
Bliss body	ANANDA MAYA	Bliss, joy, intelligence, wisdom Equates with Sattva Interpenetrates all previous sheaths Only experienced in a state of enlightenment or higher stages of meditative practice (Dhyana)

Like a tapestry, the KOSHA are interwoven layers. You have no doubt experienced this in your own body: When you are tense or strained, your breath becomes shallow, your mind becomes easily agitated, and wisdom and joy seem far away. When you are filled with joy and communion with life, these feelings permeate your entire being. Separating the strands of the tapestry is a way to look at how your whole being can become integrated or in discord.

The Art of Journaling

Aside from keeping a Teaching Journal, the art of journalling is a therapeutic brain dump and can serve as a light into your dark, unexplored recesses of your mind.

- I like using sturdy, journals that are nice to the touch! Some people use an app on their mobile phone. You may wish to journal on your computer. Whatever you choose, make it yours. Let it reflect who you are and make sure it works with your lifestyle; otherwise, you will stop.

- Write when you can, ideally at a regular time in the day. It is starting a new habit like brushing your teeth. Some people like to write first thing when they wake up, before their conscious mind creeps into the writing. Some like to do it before bed. I write after my yoga practice and before bedtime.

- You can doodle, make lists, draw a mind map, ask questions, etc. There is no right or wrong way to journal, and if you are new to journalling, take time to nurture this new habit. It does not matter if it is one word, or if you write pages. Through your scribbles, you will be able to explore patterns, observe your fears and gain a deeper understanding of yourself.

- If you are stuck on what to write, here are some questions to prompt you:

  - How are you feeling?

  - How was your practice today?

  - Are you becoming too comfortable with your practice?

  - Are you happy with your life right now?

  - What are some things you are grateful for today?

  - Did you learn anything today?

  - Are you noticing patterns that you would like to change?

Additional Reading

Essence of the Upanishads (Wisdom of India)
Eknath Easwaran

Essence of the Bhagavad Gita (Wisdom of India)
Eknath Easwaran
Key points to enquire: The relevance of the Gita to modern day yoga

The Yoga Sutras of Patanjali
Alistair Shearer
Key points to enquire include: The mind, Klesha, Kriya Yoga, Ishvara, Siddhi, Yama, Niyama

Yoga: Reflections on the Yoga Sutras of Patanjali
Bernard Bouanchaud

Hatha Yoga Pradipika
Muktibodhananda Swami
Key points to enquire: Nadi, Chakra, Granthi, Kundalini, Kriya (including Neti, Jihva Neti, Tratakan, Kapalabhati, Nauli)

The Heart of Yoga: Developing a Personal Practice
T.K.V. Desikachar

The Yoga Tradition
Georg Feuerstein

Yoga: The Spirit and Practice of Moving Into Stillness
Eric Schiffman

Yoga for Dummies
Georg Feuerstein & Larry Payne

How Yoga Works
Geshe Michael Roach and Christie McNally

The Wisdom of Healing: A Comprehensive Guide to Ayurvedic Mind-Body Medicine
David Simon

The Key Poses of Yoga
Ray Long

www.ingramcontent.com/pod-product-compliance
Lightning Source LLC
Chambersburg PA
CBHW080756030726
47592CB00010B/2877